Tie one on:

Whether you already have a drawer full of scarfs or are going out to buy this year's fabulous styles,

Sensational Scarfs

will show you how you can create fantastic new looks with a scarf and these easy-to-follow instructions.

However you choose to wear your scarf—as a head wrap, around your neck, as a belt, or as a halter—once you start you won't leave home without one.

Sensational SCARFS

44

*Great Ways
to Turn a
Scarf into
a Fabulous
Fashion Look*

Carol Straley

THREE RIVERS PRESS • NEW YORK

Published by Three Rivers Press, New York, New York.
Member of the Crown Publishing Group.

Random House, Inc. New York, Toronto, London, Sydney, Auckland
www.randomhouse.com

THREE RIVERS PRESS is a registered trademark and the Three
Rivers Press colophon is a trademark of Random House, Inc.

Originally published as a Prince Paperback in 1985.

Printed in the United States of America

Design by Mercedes Everett

Library of Congress Cataloging-in-Publication Data
is available upon request.

ISBN 0-517-88616-2

20 19

Contents

We gratefully acknowledge the editorial assistance given to us by the people at Echo Scarfs. Echo Scarfs has been a leader in the design and creation of scarfs and fashion accessories since 1923. Their products can be found at 4,000 fine stores in the United States and in Canada.

Introduction

scarf is more than an afterthought, something you knot at the neck before you run out the door. A scarf can be the eye-catching extra that gives anything you wear a fabulous finish. It can add polish, pull together an outfit, or be the main attraction. With a collection of scarfs you have everything you need to invent exciting new fashions by the dozen—if you know how to use them.

That's what this book is all about. It shows you all the different ways to twist and tie, loop and knot, and wrap and sash a scarf. There are looks for work and for weekends. In seconds the neat stack of scarfs on your shelf can become slouchy double-wrap belts, dashing menswear ties, sexy bandeau tops, evening wraps, cover-ups for swim suits, hair accessories, and more.

On these pages you'll find simple step-by-step instructions that make scarf dressing a snap. Even if you're all thumbs now, this book will have you wrapping up great new looks with ease in no time. And to help your scarf savvy there are tips on coordinating colors, mixing pattern and texture, what scarfs to collect, and how to keep your scarfs in good-as-new condition.

Once you master the basics you'll want to go on to create your own one-of-a-kind fashions. In fact, you may never get dressed again without reaching for a scarf!

Building a Basic Scarf Wardrobe

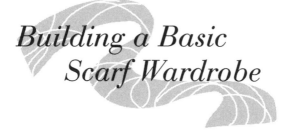

With the right scarfs at your fingertips there's no end to the number of great looks you can come up with. Your styling options depend on the shapes and sizes of the scarfs you own. Here's what to collect:

— *Ties*: tubular ties and bias ties for dapper menswear neckties and floppy bow ties

— *Squares*: 15" × 24" squares to tie at the neck or wear as head wraps, hair accessories

> • 27" × 30" squares work as belts and sashes, bikini tops, and head wraps
> • 36" × 45" squares make perfect halter tops and shoulder wraps
> • 54" × 60" squares can be tossed over your shoulders as a shawl, tied as a skirt, or wrapped as a sarong

— *Oblongs*: easy to wrap as mufflers, belts, bows, and ascots; invest in oversized oblongs to fling over one should of a dress or jacket and anchor with a belt

A word about prints: To strike the right eye-catching balance, the bigger the scarf, the bolder the pattern can be. Buy smaller scarfs in smaller prints.

Quality counts. A good scarf can last a lifetime so it pays to buy the best you can afford. When shopping always hold the scarf by the corner to see how it falls. The fabric should be soft and supple for easy handling. And give it the tie test: knot two ends. Does the scarf tie easily or does it bunch up? Don't buy the scarf unless it promises to perform beautifully in your hands.

Color Code

Whenever you put together a scarf look, consider color. The way you color-coordinate your scarfs with your clothes can add up to instant impact. When buying anything from a tie to a sarong take your pick from the three basic color groups:

Brash Brights

Shades run the spectrum from brilliant jewel tones—turquoise, emerald, topaz, garnet —to high-voltage neon colors —electric blue, shocking pink, hot yellow. Scarfs in bright colors give a fresh burst of energy to clothes in black, white, cream, gray, or navy. Or for extra sizzle try a bright on-bright effect, a sunshine-yellow scarf with a rich amethyst jacket, or a bold blue waist wrap cinching a racy red dress.

Delicate Pastels

Pale, pretty shades that look like misty watercolors have an irresistibly feminine appeal. Try apricot, melon, peach, seashell pink, lavender. For a soft, sophisticated effect pair a pastel scarf with clothes in muted neutral tones—white, beige, silver gray, camel, khaki.

Knockout Neutrals

These are the go-with-everything classics—ivory, black, gold, taupe, pearl gray, slate blue, sand, terra cotta, cinnamon. What to wear with scarfs in neutral tones? Anything goes—brights, pastels, and other neutrals.

Prints for Pizzazz

From small houndstooth checks to splashy floral designs, prints give scarfs more eye appeal. And today there are patterns galore: madras, crisp and clean geometrics, exotic paisleys, racing checks, free-form abstract designs, traditional tartan plaids, and more.

Now putting a print scarf with a solid-toned blouse is basic, but it's not the only way to go. For more individual style try these unexpected pattern mixes:

> • A tie splashed with navy and white dots with a navy-and-white striped shirt
> • A bold black-and-white floral print ascot with a black-and-white houndstooth jacket
> • A skinny-striped muffler in gray and pink with a big-plaid gray-and-pink blazer
> • A blue-and-cream diagonal-striped waist wrap with a blue-and-cream vertical-striped dress

What makes these combinations work? The colors in the pattern of the scarf are an even match with the colors in the patterns of the clothes. Experiment. Just keep in mind that the scale of the pattern of the scarf shouldn't overpower the pattern of your clothes.

Texture–Inviting to the Touch

Texture offers visual contrast, an extra dimension that you can feel as well as see. Think of nubby cotton knits, the liquid shimmer of flowing silk, the airy look of open-weave rayon. To take style one step further, coordinate the texture of your scarfs with the texture of your clothes:

> • Wear a romantic, frothy lace scarf with a rough-and-tumble denim jacket.
> • Use a soft, sensuous silk wrap with a crisp linen dress.
> • Tie a crinkled cotton mesh scarf at the waist of a flat-knit cotton dress.
> • Try floaty silk chiffon woven with golden metallic thread over a raw silk top.

Any number of textures are compatible. The idea: go for contrasts, complements, a play of one distinctive texture against another.

How to Fold a Scarf

Your first step in wrapping up any number of fashion looks is folding your scarf in one of three basic shapes: bias, triangle, or oblong. Most of the fashions in this book are based on these three patterns.

Bias

Place a square on a flat surface, wrong side up, so that it forms a diamond. Bring the top and bottom points to meet in the center. Fold the top of the scarf down to make it as wide or slim as you want.

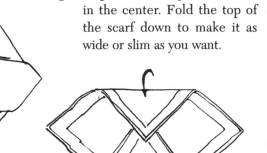

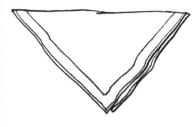

Triangle

Take a square and fold the points to meet in a triangle.

Oblong

To fold a square into an oblong, place it flat, wrong side up. Fold the top edge toward you and the opposite edge away from you. Keep folding the scarf until it is as wide as you want it.

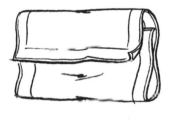

To make an oblong scarf slimmer, place on a flat surface. Fold the top and bottom edges toward the center. Keep folding the scarf in this way until it is the width you want.

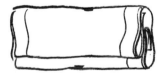

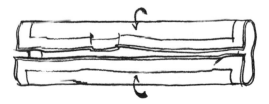

Basic Looks from Basic Folding How-Tos

Going from a basic folding technique to a finished style is a snap. Here are three classics you'll want to try.

Whimsical Windsor-knotted Scarf

Fold a square into a triangle. Place it on your shoulders with the point in back. Flip the right end over the left and tie. Next, bring the left end over the right and tie. Last, adjust the knot in front and let the ends fall freely.

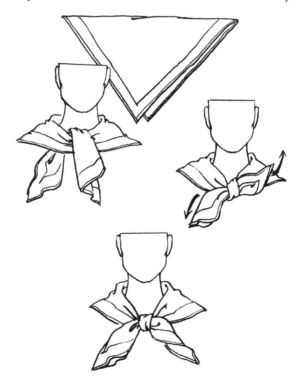

Double-wrapped Collar

Fold a square scarf on the bias. Start from the front and wrap the scarf twice around your neck. Pull ends back to front. Flip the ends over one another and slide to one side.

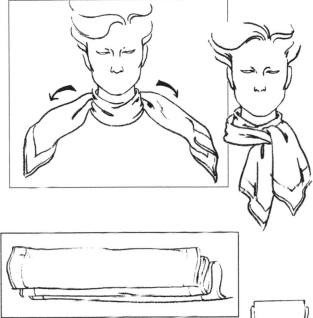

Elegant Ascot

Fold a square into an oblong or fold an oblong to make it narrower. Knot around your neck once. Flip one end over the other and smooth out both ends to make them fuller. For extra polish, tuck into an open neckline.

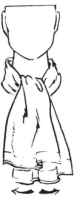

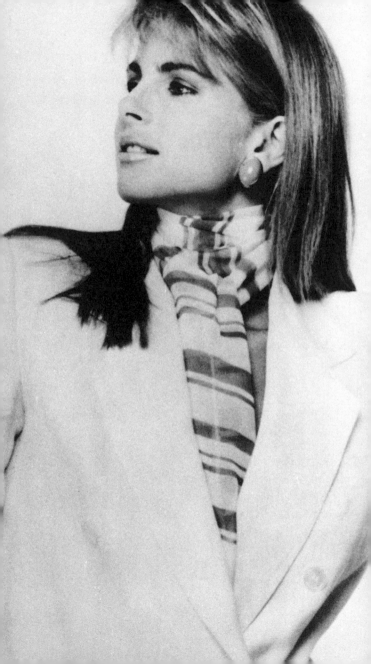

Neckline
Accents

Simply sophisticated. Tuck a soft-collar version of the classic ascot into the neckline of a jacket. Wrapped right up to the chin, the scarf also works to flatter the shape of your face.

Take an oblong scarf; starting from the front wrap it twice around your neck, then bring the ends to the front. Cross the ends; flip the end that's on top under, then over the loop. Tug gently to secure.

Country Classic

Fold a long scarf into an oblong, then fold it in half. Take the folded end in one hand, then the two loose ends with the other hand, and place at the back of the neck.

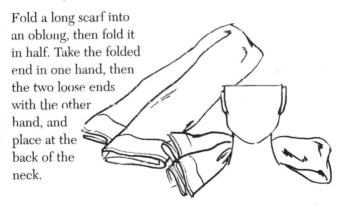

Pull the two ends through the loop of the folded end. Next, pull ends in the opposite direction until the scarf fits snugly around your neck.

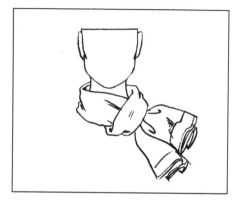

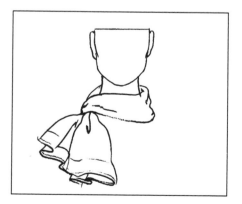

Cowboy Chic

Bring a style from the Wild West up to the minute. Fold a large square scarf into a triangle. Place low under your collarbone with the point over to one side rather than smack down the middle. Tie the ends over the opposite shoulder.

Soft Fan Collar

A flirty style. Fold a long scarf into an oblong. Wrap it twice around your neck, leaving one end longer than the other. Loop the ends over each other, then pull the longer end half-way through and work into a soft, puffy shape.

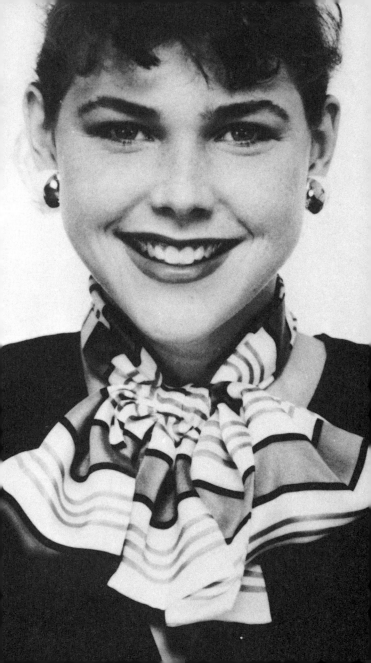

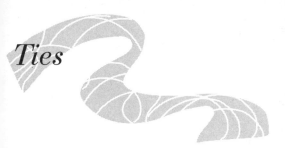

Ties

Nothing dresses up a simple sweater or jacket faster than a full, fluffy bow, easy to knot and loop with a tubular tie.

To tie a fluffy bow, place a 5″ × 54″ tubular tie around your neck so that the left end is shorter than the right. Wrap the left end around the right. Make one half of a bow with

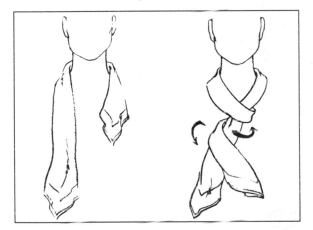

the top end and wrap the opposite end around the bow from left to right. Tuck the loose ends through the loop to make the other half of the bow. Pull both ends of the bow to shorten them until you get a full, fluffed-out shape.

Here's a dashing look borrowed from the boys, a classic necktie. Place a tie under the collar of a shirt or blouse so that the left end is shorter than the right. Wrap the right

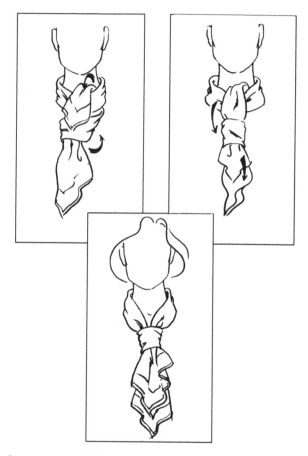

end twice around the left. Pull the long end up through the V shape at the top of the tie, then pull down through the loop. Holding the left end in the left hand, push the knot up with the right hand.

Inspired by a snappy sailor's uniform, a nautical middy tie gives a white shirt shipshape style. And because it draws the eye downward, it gives the illusion of a longer neck. Loop and knot a long tubular tie or a bias tie like a man's necktie. Slide the knot to the middle of the tie and let the ends fall freely.

A pretty style for evening. Wrap a bias tie around the waist. Make a soft, fluttery bow to one side— very feminine

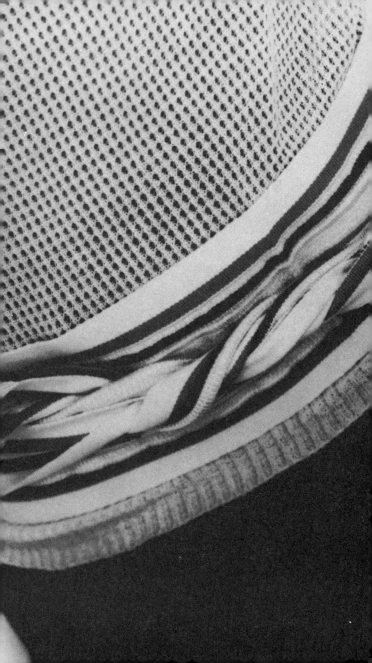

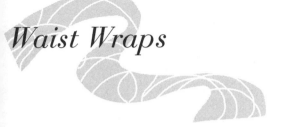

Waist Wraps

A sleek, svelte look with a new twist: cinch a pullover top or dress at the waist with a double-wrapped scarf.

Place the center of an extra-long scarf across the front of your body at the waist. Bring the ends behind you, cross them, then twist and bring to the front. Knot and tuck in the ends.

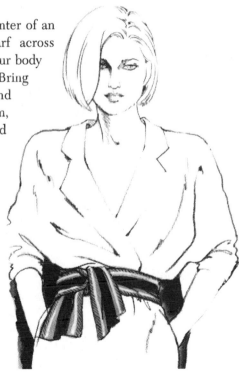

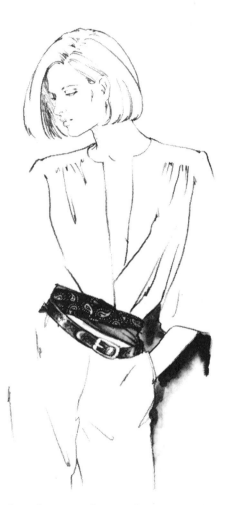

Double the fun of waist-sashing. Take two extra-long scarfs, one in a jazzy print, the other in a solid tone. Double-wrap each around the waist. Tie the ends of the first scarf in a bow; twist the ends of the second scarf. For more impact, add a loose belt slung low at the hips.

Very provocative: a sash wrapped low at the hip over a body-skimming knit dress. Place an extra-long scarf or sash at the hips in back. Bring the ends in front, cross them, twist, then bring the ends in back and tie a knot to one side.

Look slimmer in seconds: hold one end of an extra-long scarf at your left side. Wrap the other end clockwise over your waist twice. Tuck the second end into the sash so that it falls softly over your right hip.

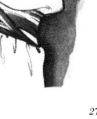

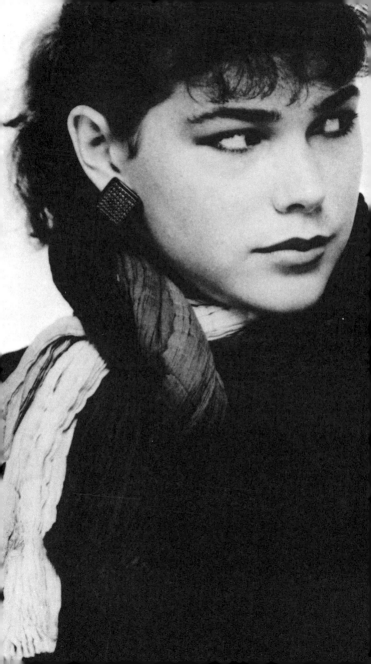

Multiple Scarf Dressing

Triple twist. For a pretty play of color and texture around the face, three scarfs are better than one. Try this look over a simple tunic top or over bare skin when you wear a strapless sundress.

Layer three 41" × 66" oblong scarfs together. Wrap once or twice around your neck. Knot and let the ends fall freely. Hint: choose scarfs that are crinkly soft but with lots of body. Good choices: pleated cotton or a cotton/linen knit.

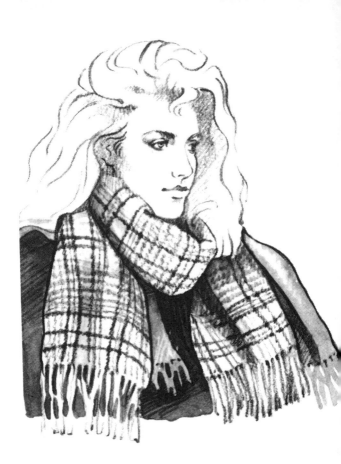

Double-take on Flair

Fold an extra-long oblong in half, lengthwise. Starting from the front, wrap ends around your neck, cross in back, and flip ends over your shoulders in front. Then take a second scarf in a contrasting color or pattern and wrap it in the same way as the first. This layered look gives you a pretty play of color and texture.

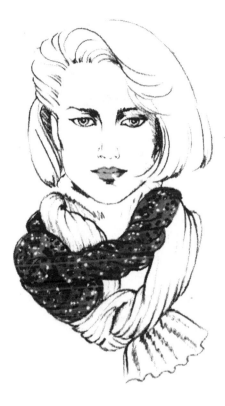

Softwear Necklace

Take two twistable scarfs, one in a print and one in a solid
color. Twist and knot the solid-color scarf in a wide circle
around your neck, leaving the end short; pull into a fan
shape. Then twist the print scarf in the same way, layering
it over the solid-color scarf and knotting the ends higher.
Instant individual style!

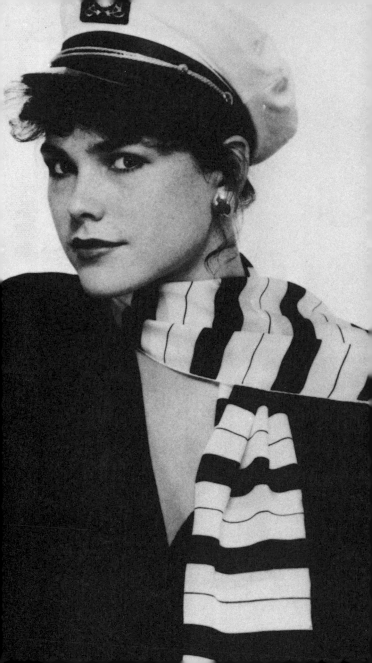

Soft Flings

Easy does it. For instant chic, place a long silk crepe scarf around your neck, then flip one end over your shoulder. Optional: secure with a gold or silver pin at the shoulder.

A New Slant

Fold an over-sized square scarf into a triangle. Drape the scarf over one shoulder so that the point falls over the arm. Knot the ends at the opposite hip and adjust the scarf so that it falls on a diagonal from shoulder to hip.

Crossover Style

Take an oversized square and fold on the bias. Fling over one shoulder so that the front falls on a slant across your body with the ends below the opposite hip. Cinch with a belt at the waist.

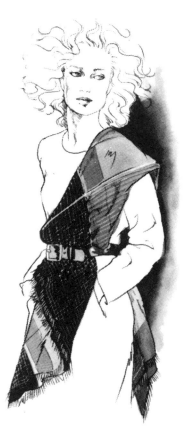

Over-the-Shoulder Fling

Toss an oversized oblong scarf over one shoulder. Adjust the scarf so that it falls over the top of your sleeve. To secure, belt the scarf at the waist and pull into a soft blouson shape for a flattering effect.

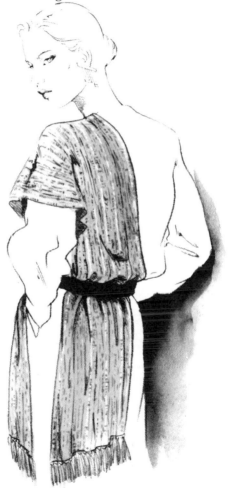

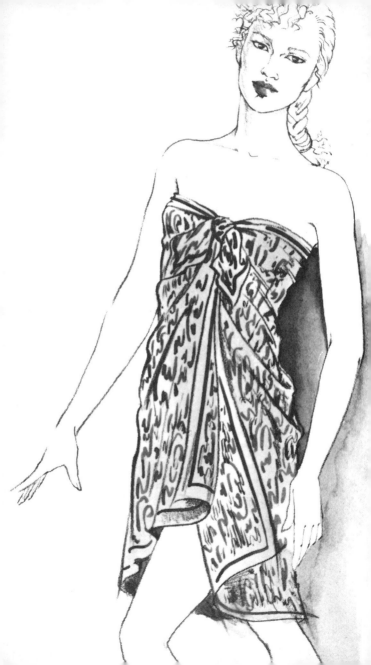

Sun Wraps

Pretty pareo. After swimming, tie on the coolest cover-up under the sun. The *pareo*, an enormous 54″ square, is ready to wrap into a sexy sarong-style dress.

Hold the pareo horizontally and place it across your back. Bring the ends under your arms to meet in front. Tie a square knot in the center. Easy!

Sarong Skirt

An easy, elegant look for evening, perfect with a sensuous silk shirt. Take a pareo and hold it horizontally behind you at the waist. Bring the ends to the front and knot securely below the waist.

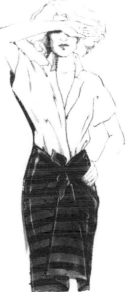

Suit Up for Sunning

Starting in front, hold a pareo vertically. Fold the top to
make a cuff; knot the ends in back. Slip between your legs
from front to back. Roll up the rest of the pareo in back. Tie
the ends around your waist and knot in front.

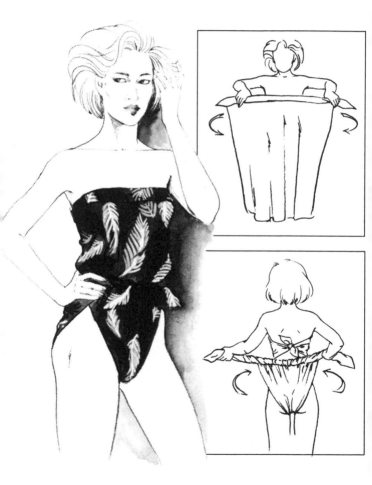

Summer Cooler

Beat the heat in an exotic wrap-and-tuck pareo. Holding the pareo horizontally, place one end under your right arm. Bring the opposite end across the front of your body to the back and then around to the front, overlapping the right end. Tuck the loose end inside the top of the pareo. If nec-essary, use a safety pin to hold the pareo in place.

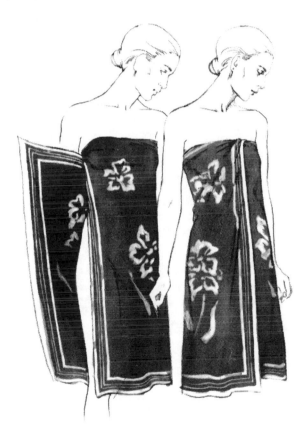

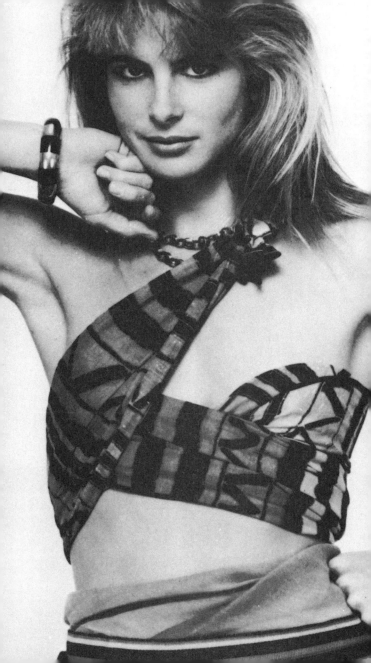

Cool Looks
for Hot Days

A beach bandeau is sensational over a tan. Scarfs sashed at the waist and hips over a summer skirt or shorts wrap up the wild, jungle look.

To tie up a bandeau, take an extra-long cotton scarf (12″ × 78″) and hold it across your back, bringing the ends under your arms. The end in your left hand should be longer than the end in your right. Bring the left end over to the right to cover bust, then cross the end in your right hand over your left shoulder. Bring the left end up to meet it and knot the scarf just below the shoulder. Next, wrap your waist with an 18″ × 71″ cotton gauze scarf; accent hips with a double-wrap sash.

Take the plunge in a sexy halter top, perfect for catching a few rays, or a poolside party. You'll need two large silk or cotton squares that are at least 27″ in diameter. Place each one in a diamond shape next to each other. Knot the triangle points that meet in the center just under breasts. Knot the two top corners behind your neck; knot the remaining corners tightly in back. Tuck any excess under.

Quick Bikini Top

Fold and wrap an 11″ × 54″ oblong scarf around your midriff into a bandeau and knot in the back. Then take a 9″ × 56″ bias scarf, loop it through the center of the bandeau in front and tie it halter style around your neck.

Wrap-Around Halter

Take a large silk or cotton square and tie the opposite points in a knot to form a triangle. Slip over your head so that the knot is behind your neck. Bring both of the bottom corners around the midriff and tie in the back.

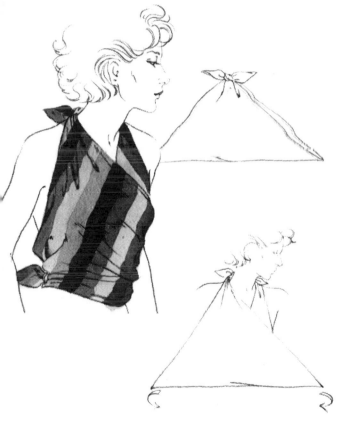

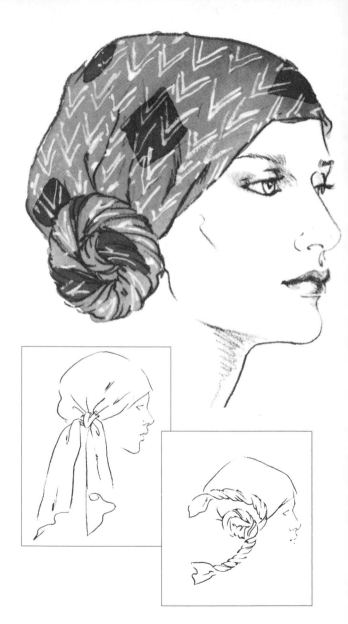

Head Wraps

A romantic wrap. Protect your hair from wind, sun, or rain with a head scarf that is finished with a soft wrap-and-tie rosette.

Fold a large square into a triangle or oblong. Place it on your head so that both ends fall over one ear. Knot the ends. Next, twist one end tightly. Coil it around the knot and tuck in the end. Do the same with the other loose end. To keep the rosette in place, slip in a few bobby pins underneath.

Gypsy Wrap

Fold a large square into a triangle. Place it on your head so that the front dips low on the forehead. Pull the ends back and knot over the point of the triangle. For a softer look, make the scarf fuller by gently pulling it above the knot.

Braided Gypsy

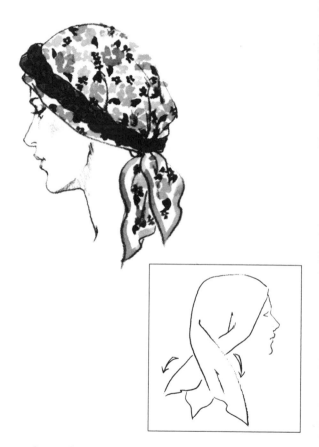

Wrap and tie a large square into the gypsy style described on the previous page. Next, take three squares, knot together, and work into a braid. Slip the braid over the scarf and knot the ends low in the back at the nape of your neck.

Triangle Turban

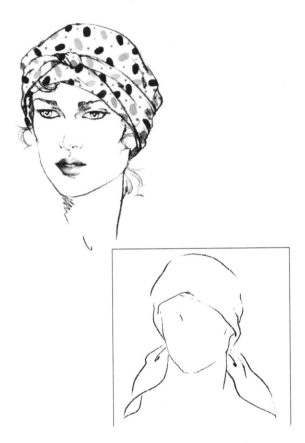

Fold a large square into a triangle. Place the scarf on your head with the point of the triangle in back. Cross the ends over the point. Bring the ends back to the front, knot above the edge of the scarf, and tuck them in.

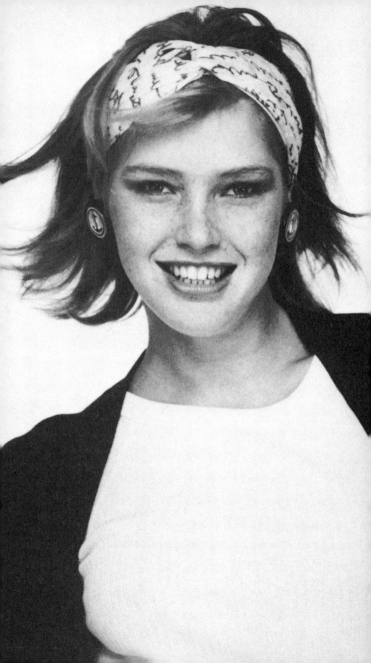

Hair Accessories

With a knot and a twist, a pretty scarf gives you an easy way to keep your hair up and away from your face, a wonderful summer standby.

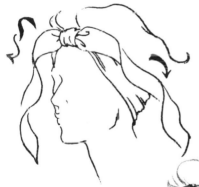

Fold an oblong or square scarf on the bias. Brush hair behind ears. Place the scarf under your hair in back, bring the ends to the front, and knot low on your forehead. Twist the loose ends tightly and tuck them under the sides.

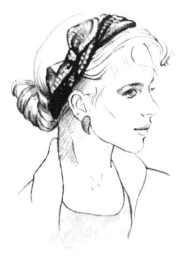

Soft control for a sleek chignon. Pull hair into a ponytail, secure with a coated elastic, and coil into a smooth knot. Slip an oblong or square scarf under the chignon, bring the ends to the front, and tie into a bow. Last, slide the bow to one side for an asymmetrical accent.

Great in a heat wave, a slouchy bandana. Place a 64"-long oblong scarf just above your eyebrows and wrap around your head to the back. Cross the ends, bring them toward the front, and knot on the sides or in front.

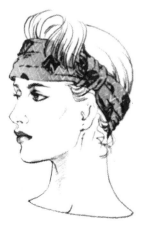

Crisscross Turban

A 64"-long oblong scarf does the trick. Start wrapping the scarf from the back, twisting the ends around each other twice. The fit should be snug but comfortable.

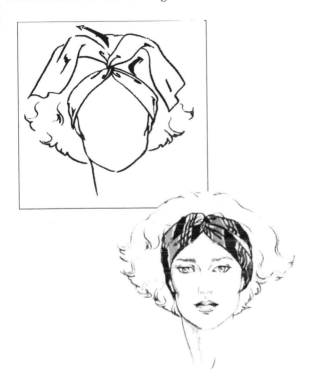

Bring the ends to the back and knot them. You can also tuck them in for a smoother look.

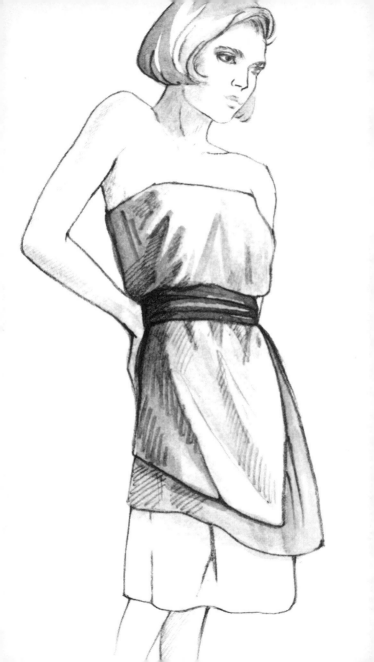

Instant
Dress-Ups

How to be ready for a night out in a flash: wrap a sarong over a silky skirt, cinch the waist with a tie.

Take a silk sarong or a 54″ square scarf and hold both ends behind you. Next, pull the sarong taut as you wrap it around you. Bring the ends to meet under one arm and knot. Blouse the top half and belt at the waist with a silk tie knotted in back.

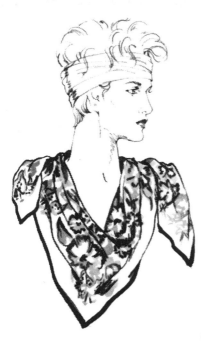

A quick way to give an A.M. look P.M. glamour. Fold a large silk scarf into a triangle. Place with the point of the triangle in front. Pull down gently to make a V neck. Cross the ends in back and then flip them over your shoulders in front. Let the ends fall freely.

Perfect for parties, a sexy halter. Take a 27″ or 31″ square scarf and fold diagonally. Tie a tiny knot where the triangle points meet. Slip a skinny gold choker through the knot and fasten it around your neck. Knot the scarf low in back.

Speedy Sash

Any dress goes from day to night with a scarf double-wrapped at the waist. Go for a touch of glitter with a scarf shot with shimmering Lurex. Starting in front, place an extra-long scarf at the waist. Wrap ends to the back, cross, and bring to the front. Tie in a big beautiful bow.

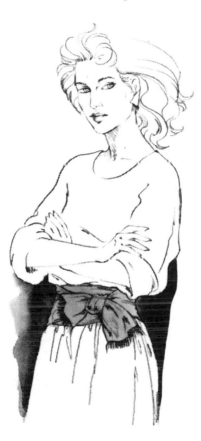

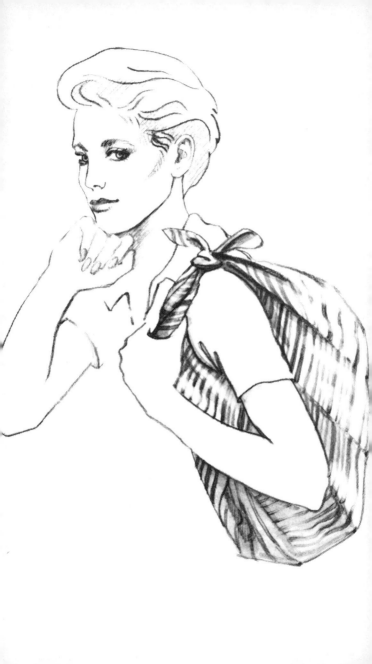

Scarf Tips and Tricks

Bag it. Turn a square scarf into a soft catch-and-carry-all. Try silk or shimmering satin for a smashing evening bag, a bright cotton scarf for a beach tote.

Spread out a 36" square on a flat surface and put what you want to carry in the middle. Take the four corners and knot together into a soft pouch.

Collar Wrap

Stand up the collar of a silk shirt. Loop a silk bias tie around your neck and add a glittery pin. Let one end of the collar flip over the scarf for a casually chic finish.

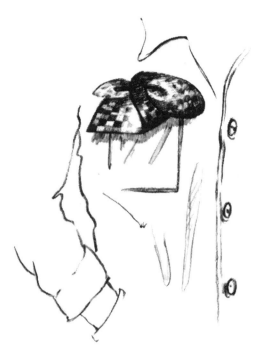

Pocket Accent

Add more dash to a classic blazer. Fold a 12″ square scarf into an oblong and tuck it into the pocket. Pull the top half that peeks out of the pocket into pretty folds.

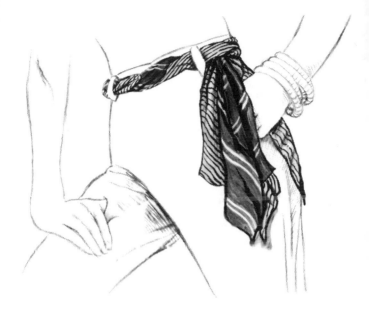

Bias Belt

Take two bias ties in contrasting yet complementary patterns and twist together. Slip through the belt loops of a pair of pants or a skirt. Knot the ends securely to one side. Super!

Tips for
Easy Care

The best way to keep your scarfs looking their best is to have them dry-cleaned. This is especially important for scarfs made of delicate fabric such as silk. Check the label for the manufacturer's care instructions. If hand-washing is an option, use a cold-water detergent made for fine washable fabrics.

Soak each scarf separately in cold water. Squeeze suds through gently. After rinsing, blot excess moisture with a towel—never ring or twist. Spread on a flat surface to dry and smooth out wrinkles.

When pressing a scarf between wearings, iron it on the "wrong" side. Use a dry iron for silk since steam can cause water-spotting.

To keep your scarfs wrinkle-free when packed for travel, try this suitcase-survival trick. Simply fold and stash each scarf in an individual plastic bag. The plastic traps air which minimizes creasing.

Instead of stuffing your scarfs in a drawer, keep them handy and ready to wear. Stack your scarfs folded in small cardboard boxes covered with pretty fabric and place on an open shelf or on top of a bureau. Or show them off in open wire baskets. You can also make your scarfs part of the decor of your room—just hang them on tie racks or Lucite bars. The array of colors and patterns will liven up the walls and your scarfs will always be within easy reach.